ERECTILE DYSFUNCTION GUIDEBOOK: THE COMPLETE SEXUAL HEALTH SOLUTION TO IDENTIFYING, WORKING ON AND CURING ED AND IMPOTENCE

Natural Remedies, Psychology, Sex Addiction, Exercise, Diet and More

DAVID WHITEHEAD

INTRODUCTION

Studies show that Erectile Dysfunction is a common condition in males between the ages of 40 to 70 years old. However, it is worth noting that just because something is common does not mean it is natural.

This book is designed to help you solve the issue of Erectile Dysfunction, evaluating every possible cause of the condition to see which course of action would work best for your situation. Taking into account not just medical but also psychological issues, this book attempts to cover all bases to help you or a loved one overcome impotence.

By the end of this book, we hope that you have sufficient information to pursue an Erectile Dysfunction treatment, whether at home or through the input of a doctor. Not only that, but this book follows a comprehensive pattern that addresses not just erectile dysfunction as a possible symptom of a worse condition – but the underlying condition itself.

Having said that, let's get down to understanding what Erectile Dysfunction is!

1

WHAT IS ERECTILE DYSFUNCTION?

Erectile dysfunction or ED is a health concern common among men who are 50 years old or more. As the term implies, the problem is distinguished by an inability to sustain an erection, or whether an erection occurs, it is often flaccid and therefore incapable of penetration.

Such can be a huge problem for men, and while the older generation tends to simply accept this condition, the fact is that erectile dysfunction need not be permanent. This book is specially designed to provide in-depth insight on erectile dysfunction, why it happens, and what could be done to resolve the problem.

DEFINING ERECTILE DYSFUNCTION

The truth is that men suffer from erectile dysfunction from time to time. This should not be a cause for concern because a man's ability to perform can vary depending on the environment, time of day, current mood, and a variety of other factors. However, suppose your inability to achieve or maintain an erection has become so prevalent that it has affected your sexual life. In that case, there's a good chance that the condition can now be diagnosed as Erectile Dysfunction.

For the most part, however, ED is best diagnosed by a doctor since there's really no exact number of days or frequency that establishes ED. A physician must perform a test to truly determine if there is an issue and, if that's the case, how to best address the problem.

What you should understand, however, is that ED is usually a symptom rather than the problem itself. Hence, males who suffer from erectile dysfunction typically have an underlying condition that affects their performance in bed. Most of the time, addressing such a problem will help fight ED, allowing males to once again achieve or maintain an erection sufficient for penetration.

HOW AN ERECTION OCCURS

Before further discussing erectile dysfunction, it's important to first find out exactly why an erection occurs. For the most part, erectile dysfunction is an interruption in one of the several processes that lead to an erection.

Arousal comes first triggered by either brain activity or any contact with the penis. When arousal occurs, the muscles of the penis relax, the blood vessels starting to expand as the blood rushes into the organ. This causes the penis to increase in size and girth until no more space is available for the blood to rush into.

With erectile dysfunction, the problem usually occurs in the blood-filling stage. Either no blood is rushing in to fill the vessels, or there is not enough blood to cause the penis to harden. Either way, it would be near-impossible for the male to successfully penetrate the vagina with the flaccid erection, causing frustration on both male and female.

ERECTILE DYSFUNCTION SYMPTOMS

The symptoms of erectile dysfunction aren't exactly complex. For the most part, there are three symptoms associated with the condition:

- You have a hard time getting an erection
- You have a hard time maintaining an erection
- Your desire for sexual activity is greatly reduced

If you notice any of these three on a prevalent or persistent basis, chances are you are suffering from erectile dysfunction. Some men think that this is a natural part of growing older and should not be a cause for concern.

As previously mentioned, however, erectile dysfunction can be a sign of an underlying health problem such as diabetes or heart issues. That being said, it's never a good idea to ignore the condition – especially if you're suffering from symptoms other than ED.

Be honest with your doctor, and don't be afraid to bring this up again the next time you go in for a checkup.

RISKS ASSOCIATED WITH ERECTILE DYSFUNCTION

More than 30 million men in America suffer from ED, as determined by the National Institute of Diabetes and Digestive and Kidney Diseases. According to the same study, 17% of men in their 60s will experience this condition, while more than 50% of men will have ED by the time they hit 75 years of age.

Understand, though, that ED is not inevitable. For the most part, the condition is dictated by the health of a man. Hence, a healthy male will most likely still function upon reaching his 70s, although, of course, attaining an erection may no longer be as easy as it used to.

Other erectile dysfunction risks include pre-existing health problems, including cardiovascular diseases, diabetes, high blood pressure, low blood pressure, and more. These will be discussed later in great detail.

ERECTILE DYSFUNCTION COMPLICATIONS

The problem with ED is that once it occurs, it leaves a deeply psychological mark that only gets worse every time. Hence, every time you suffer from erectile dysfunction, the stress and anxiety pile on so that you start to convince yourself you will never have an erection again. Complications arising from ED include but are not limited to the following:

- Stress and anxiety
- Unsatisfactory sex life
- Problems with the relationship
- Low self-esteem
- Difficulty or inability in getting your partner pregnant

DIAGNOSING ERECTILE DYSFUNCTION AND MEETING WITH YOUR DOCTOR

Since there are lots of possible reasons for erectile dysfunction, visiting the doctor will include lots of questions on both your parts. It's crucial that your physician asks as many questions as possible to determine the most probable cause of your ED. Below are some pointers to keep in mind as you plan your visit:

- Make a list of all the symptoms you've had
- Try to take note of any defining moments in the past days or weeks that you feel your doctor should know
- • Before making an appointment, inquire in advance about what you can do. A blood test, for example, may be required by the doctor. If this is the case, you may need to fast for 8 hours to obtain an accurate reading.
- List down all the medications you're currently using and how often
- Your diet, exercise regimen, and supplement used should also be listed down as they may influence erectile dysfunction
- If possible, bring your partner with you. This should make it easier for the doctor to determine certain factors relating to the ED.

When visiting the doctor, there's just one simple rule to always follow: NEVER LIE. Embarrassment should be kicked out as you provide your doctor with only the most basic facts regarding your condition. You never know what factors could be contributory to your condition, so do not hold anything back.

OTHER MALE SEXUAL DYSFUNCTIONS

Note that erectile dysfunction is different from other male sexual dysfunctions, such as premature or delayed ejaculation. In these cases, there is sufficient erection for successful penetration. However, the male usually ejaculates too early or too soon, causing dissatisfaction on the part of the female.

Premature/delayed ejaculation stems from other health

issues that require somewhat similar treatment. For the purpose of this book, however, we'll focus mostly on erectile dysfunction, its causes, and how to treat the condition.

THE CAUSES OF ERECTILE DYSFUNCTION

As previously mentioned, erectile dysfunction can be caused by several issues, the most prominent of which is age. You'll find, however, that many young men also suffer from the condition due to lifestyle issues. Suppose you suffer from erectile dysfunction or want to avoid or treat the condition completely. In that case, the following are some factors that can affect your performance in bed: Heart Disease, Obesity, Diabetes, Clogged Arteries, High Blood Pressure, etc.

Heart Disease

Any problem with the heart results in an insufficient amount of blood being pumped into the body. As most people know, blood carries all the important nutrients and minerals all over the system, giving crucial life to every organ in the body. Heart disease, therefore, makes it nearly impossible for the muscle to pump fast enough or strong enough to distribute blood to every portion of the body – including the penis. That being said, even when a person is aroused and the blood vessels expand, there's not enough blood pumped inside said vessels, resulting in a flaccid erection. In cases like this, the heart problem and the ED itself must be addressed using healthy living and specific medications.

Obesity

Obesity interferes with practically each body process, so it stands to reason that it can affect the capacity to obtain or maintain an erection. For the most part, obesity squeezes the blood vessels, making it difficult for the blood to go through all parts of the body. Don't forget the fact that obesity expands the body, and in most cases, the heart finds it difficult to pump sufficient amounts of blood all over the system – especially towards the penis. The additional layer of fat lying on the heart also makes it difficult for the heart to pump blood, thereby restricting its overall capacity. All in all, obesity presents an array of situations that could affect the capacity to obtain an erection.

Diabetes

Diabetes is often a problem with the blood itself. Since the condition causes a thickening of the blood, the normal flow through the veins is compromised. Imagine a thick and syrupy consistency flowing through the veins rather than a watery consistency – chances are the 'syrup' would flow slower than the latter.

Clogged Arteries

Clogged arteries triggering erectile dysfunction work

pretty much the same way as cardiovascular issues. The blockage in the arteries makes it difficult for the heart to pump blood all over the system, severely restricting the amount of blood that flows to the organs. Imagine water being pushed through a very narrow hose – no matter how high the pressure might be, the fact is that there is less water being pumped out per heartbeat.

High Blood Pressure

High blood pressure or hypertension leads to ED if the condition is left untreated for a long time. This is because hypertension manages to 'damage' the blood vessels over time as the blood rushes through the vessels at such a high force.

This can cause problems to every body part where blood vessels can be found – including the penis. Once the ability of the vessels to retain blood becomes compromised, it becomes more difficult for males to attain or maintain an erection.

Substance Abuse

Both drug and alcohol misuse can cause erectile dysfunction because they constrict blood vessels and render it harder for fluid to enter the penis. Note that the keyword here is 'abuse,' which can be characterized by continuous drinking well beyond the legal limit. Males who are binge drinkers may suffer from erectile dysfunction even when they're sober. The same holds for those who use drugs.

Smoking

Smoking is also another huge risk factor when it comes to ED. It manages to affect erection in the same way as alcohol –

by constricting the blood vessels so that they have a hard time fully filling the penis. Each stick of cigarette increases the risk of ED, although studies show that constant smokers who decide to quit manage to shake off erectile dysfunction after being clean for a certain length of time.

Depression and Other Psychological Issues

Erectile Dysfunction is also common in men who suffer from emotional or psychological issues. Stress and anxiety are the typical causes that may stem from several issues, such as relationship problems, work issues, or even the death of a loved one. It's not uncommon for widowers to suffer from erectile dysfunction months or even years after the death of their spouse.

Psychological issues resulting in erectile dysfunction are often addressed through the help of a therapist. Anti-depressant medications may be provided, but for the most part, the process is a long and slow one as the underlying condition is addressed with ED merely regarded as a symptom. Further in this book, we'll talk about how you can address the issue of depression and ED, hopefully bypassing the process of seeing a therapist for the condition.

Surgeries or Injuries

Of course, it's important to also take into account surgeries or injuries resulting in ED. For the most part, such injuries or surgeries hit certain nerves or vessels that have something to do with an erection. If the condition stems from this kind of problem, the best solution would be another surgery to correct the condition.

Sleep Issues

Insomnia or lack of sleep can be another factor for erectile dysfunction. Improper amounts of sleep over a period of time are tantamount to stress and anxiety, in most cases being a symptom of depression. If you're having sleep issues due to depression or any other psychological issue, the root cause of the problem must be addressed through the help of a professional.

Peyronie's Disease

Peyronie's Disease is a condition wherein the penis bends upwards or sideways due to a plaque buildup inside the organ. This is not an in-born condition but can happen over time – both to young and older men.

Porn in Erectile Dysfunction

Studies also show that men who constantly watch and masturbate to porn have higher chances of suffering from Erectile Dysfunction. More on this will be discussed later.

OTHER CAUSES OF ERECTILE DYSFUNCTION

- Prolonged bicycling
- Prostate cancer
- Parkinson's disease
- Some medications

With so many causes for erectile dysfunction, it stands to reason that there are also numerous ways to address the problem. In instances when erectile dysfunction is a symptom rather than the problem itself, it's crucial to treat the underlying difficulty in the hope of eventually addressing erectile dysfunction.

In the next Chapters, we'll tackle each ED cause as discussed above and provide treatment options for each situation.

3

HORMONES: A MAJOR CAUSE OF ERECTILE DYSFUNCTION

As previously mentioned, Erectile Dysfunction is not an inevitable condition and not dependent on age alone. However, it is an inarguable fact that obtaining and maintaining an erection becomes more difficult as a male reaches old age.

This is mostly attributed to the body's reduced production of hormones. Note, though, that old age is not the only possible cause of a decrease in hormone production. The following conditions may also present the same situation:

HYPOGONADISM

Thyroid problems may either be too much production of hormones or too little production of hormones. Either way, this leads to erectile dysfunction in men, which can be treated by stimulating the production of hormones or through straight-out hormone replacement therapy. Some of the symptoms of this condition in men are:

- Muscle loss

- Body hair loss
- Breast growth
- Erectile dysfunction
- Osteoporosis
- Infertility
- Fatigue
- The decreased growth of penis and testicles
- Low libido
- Hot flashes
- Difficulty concentrating

CUSHING'S SYNDROME

This is a condition in which the body releases excessive cortisol, resulting in menstrual irregularities and erectile dysfunction in men. There is no definitive test to diagnose Cushing's, but the condition has been sufficiently studied to help with treatment. The treatment itself depends on the possible cause of the condition. Following are some of the symptoms of Cushing:

- Weight gain or obesity
- Fatty deposits
- Acne
- Fatigue
- Glucose intolerance
- Decreased fertility
- Loss of interest in sex
- Thinning skin
- Anxiety and irritability
- Depression

4

DIABETES-INDUCED ERECTILE DYSFUNCTION

The only upside of having ED due to diabetes is the fact that diabetes is easy to diagnose. Many doctors today specialize in this condition, thus giving you the chance to immediately find out if you're diabetic and what can be done to stave off any health problem resulting from the condition. More often than not, erectile dysfunction is attributed to Type 2 Diabetes rather than Type 1.

What you should understand is that diabetes is not curable but treatable. This means that once diagnosed, you have to commit to a regimen that will keep your blood sugar down – typically involving a strict diet and an exercise regimen.

Here are some things to keep in mind if you have diabetes-related erectile dysfunction. Signs and Symptoms of Diabetes Contrary to popular belief, diabetic people aren't all obese or overweight. In fact, rapid weight loss is one of the symptoms of diabetes. If you notice any of the following signs alongside erectile dysfunction, chances are your blood sugar is too high:

- Excessive thirst
- Frequent urination
- Sudden and unexplained weight loss
- Blurred vision
- Difficulty concentrating
- Always being tired
- Stomach pain
- Vomiting and nausea
- Numbness in the hands and feet

Note that these symptoms don't appear all at once. For the most part, frequent urination, excessive thirst, and weight loss are the warning signs of diabetes. Should you experience these, it's best to consult your doctor immediately so that something can be done.

Note, however, that erectile dysfunction is typically a latter symptom. This means that if you're suffering from ED due to diabetes, chances are the condition is already present long-term and that you're also suffering from the other symptoms associated with this health issue. A visit to the doctor is imperative.

DIABETIC DIET

The best way to handle diabetes is through a strict diet or food regimen. Once you've been diagnosed by your doctor with this condition, it's important to get your food regimen under control. Here's what you should know about food, diabetes, and erectile dysfunction: Sugar Checks

If you come from a long line of diabetics, simply checking your blood sugar would be enough to tell you whether you're hovering in the 'danger' zone. By frequent sugar checks, you have the chance to find out if your sugar is getting too high and whether you need to be more cautious with your diet and exercise.

You should be able to perform routine sugar checks through blood meter glucose. This is available without a prescription and can be bought over the counter. They're easy enough to use and will give you accurate readings, which should signify the following:

- 100 mg/dL or below – normal
- 100 to 120 mg/dL – probably pre-diabetes; if this is your reading, then your chances of suffering from diabetes within the next five years is higher. This is the best time to do something about the condition, preferably sticking to a healthy diet and exercise routine. However, at this stage, it's unlikely that any erectile dysfunction you have can be attributed to diabetes or pre-diabetes.
- 126 mg/dL or more – this is a likely indicator of diabetes. If your sugar reading is within this mark, the chances are that diabetes is a contributory factor, if not the major factor to your erectile dysfunction. If this is the case, you will have to address the condition by treating the diabetes.
- 200 mg/dL or more – two random tests resulting in a 200 mg/dL reading is diagnostically considered verification for diabetes. Your erectile dysfunction is highly likely to be the result of your diabetic status.

Note that you can't check your blood sugar at any time of the day. If you've just eaten, then your blood sugar will read higher than normal. That being said, individuals are often advised to fast for eight straight hours before a blood check.

This includes coffee or any kind of drink except water. If your blood glucose readings are high, consult your doctor to follow up with what could be done.

DIET FOR DIABETES AND ERECTILE DYSFUNCTION

It logically follows that if diabetes is the root cause of your ED, you should follow a diabetes-specific diet. As already mentioned, diabetes is not curable, but it is treatable. Here's how food should be approached if you have ED and Diabetes.

Carbohydrates High in Fiber with Slow Release

A low-carbohydrate diet is typically suggested for diabetics, but this ruling isn't absolute. High fiber carbohydrates providing a slow release of energy is best because it doesn't spike your blood sugar levels. The digestion is slower so that you'll be given a steady amount of energy during the day. Here's a rundown of common slow-release carbohydrates:

- Low-sugar bran flakes
- Whole wheat pasta
- Brown rice
- Rolled oats
- Steel-cut oats
- Leafy green vegetables

WHAT TO AVOID

It suffices to say that diabetics should avoid sugary foods and fast-release carbohydrates. Unfortunately, the list of food to avoid is infinitely longer than what you can actually eat. As a general rule, anything that comes packaged or processed should NOT be consumed by a diabetic. This includes canned food, deep-fried foods, bread, cereals, processed meat, and products that claim to be 'low fat.'

5

HEART ISSUES AND ERECTILE DYSFUNCTION

Erectile Dysfunction is a symptom of heart disease – which means that chances are you'll be suffering from ED before figuring out that you have cardiovascular issues.

HEART ISSUES AND ED

Heart problems affect the body's ability to supply blood to all body parts – including the penis. Simply put, problems with blood flow reduce the amount of blood flowing to the penis during erection, hence the inability to attain or maintain a shaft capable of penetration.

Studies have shown that there's a strong link between cardiovascular problems and erectile dysfunction. Males who are noticing ED problems or the beginning of such are advised to have their hearts checked as soon as possible.

RISK FACTORS

How do you know you have heart problems resulting from ED? An actual diagnosis of a doctor is typically the best and most accurate way of figuring this out. The good news is that the diagnosis involves non-invasive procedures that take only a few minutes to accomplish. Other causes that can raise the likelihood of cardiac complications include, but are not restricted to, the following:

- Diabetes
- Alcohol use
- Smoking
- High blood pressure
- High cholesterol
- Low testosterone
- Obesity

TREATMENT OPTIONS

The good news is that since ED is a preliminary symptom of heart disease, your steps to overcome the problem need not be extensive. There are medications that the doctor can recommend, although the most prevalent treatment is lifestyle changes. This includes restriction in your diet as well as an increase in the proper type of exercise.

Medications

Medications for heart problems are pretty prevalent and decrease the risk of heart attacks for the common male. Unfortunately, heart medications disqualify males from taking drugs for erectile dysfunction, which essentially doesn't solve the problem at all when it comes to sexual relations.

The good news is that if you are one of the males prescribed these medications, you can now ask your doctor for a different type of pill. New medications are now ED-friendly which means that you can take them WITH erectile dysfunction pills such as Viagra. Of course, it's crucial to first ask your doctor about this beforehand.

Lifestyle Changes

Generally speaking, individuals with heart problems are advised against eating fatty food items, prepackaged food, and basically anything that isn't fresh fruits and vegetables. Here's what you should know about lifestyle changes necessary to reverse heart issues:

- Maintain a healthy weight, preferably a normal one as defined by the body
- Mass Index
- Quit smoking and alcohol – another two common instances increasing the risk of ED
- Eat a healthy diet
- Get used to exercising. For heart reasons, excessive exercise is not advisable. However, walking at least 30 minutes early in the morning should contribute to heart health
- Learn to manage stress better by being part of relaxing activities. Golf is perhaps one of the best exercises today for males who suffer from heart problems.
- Learn to manage high cholesterol and high blood pressure issues

6

HOW BLOOD PRESSURE LEADS TO ERECTILE DYSFUNCTION

High blood pressure, also known as hypertension, can destroy blood arteries, reducing blood supply to various areas of the body. Therefore, this can lead to ED as the shaft doesn't get sufficient blood flow to achieve or maintain an erection. However, in a cruel twist of fate, studies show that medications used to treat high blood pressure come with side effects that can cause ED.

SYMPTOMS OF HIGH BLOOD PRESSURE

High blood pressure is called the "Silent Killer" because it is largely asymptomatic. This means that there are NO symptoms attributed to the condition, so unless you're constantly checking, there's no way to know whether you have hypertension. Instead, you'll simply be shocked at the aftereffects of the problem as it slowly damages the blood vessels in your body.

So how do you know your hypertension is the primary cause of ED? The good news is that there are devices to help with this, and they're very easy to use. Strap-on products can instantly inform you of your blood pressure for monitoring purposes.

Despite the lack of symptoms, however, there are those who swear by different signs that indicate HBP. Dizziness, blood spots in the eyes, and facial flushing are some of the indicators people go by.

RISKS OF HYPERTENSION

Although you might not notice any side effects, there are instances that put you at a much higher risk for this condition. If you fall under any of the given categories, it's best to have your blood pressure checked on a routine basis just to be sure.

MONITORING YOUR BLOOD PRESSURE

Manual reading of your blood pressure is often more accurate than a digital strap-on. It's best to learn how to use the manual reading so that you'll be more assured of the results. Either way, however, you don't want your blood pressure (BP) to be more than 120/80.

Systolic and Diastolic

Systolic refers to the top number or the highest one of the two. It measures the pressure in the arteries when the heart contracts. The diastolic pressure is the lowest and corresponds to the pressure when the heart is at rest or between beats. Now, these two numbers may vary in reading and will not always be exactly 120/80. For example, the reading might be 110 over 90 or 120 over 60. When judging your BP, it's important to look at BOTII.

Generally, a healthy blood pressure reading is one with the systolic below 120 AND diastolic below 80.

Pre Hypertension

Prehypertension is shown by systolic blood pressure readings of 120 to 139 or diastolic blood pressure readings of 80 to 89. Note that your reading may be 110 over 85 – this will still indicate hypertension even if your systolic is within normal levels. Pre-hypertension, however, is the perfect time for you to make changes in your lifestyle with the hope of eventually reversing the condition.

High Blood Pressure Stage 1

This is the status when your systolic is between 140 to 159 or if your diastolic is between 90 to 99. At this stage, it's important to make an even more conscious effort into changing your lifestyle to lower BP at more normal levels.

Consistently ranking at Stage 1 for a long amount of time is sufficient to cause damage to your blood vessels, so if you have ED, chances are you're at least in this particular stage.

High Blood Pressure Stage 2

Stage 2 starts when your systolic is higher than 160 and your diastolic higher than 100. Once you hit this stage, make every effort to lower your BP.

Hypertensive Crisis

Once your BP hits 180 or higher for systolic or if diastolic hits 110 or higher – this is an emergency crisis and necessitates a visit to the hospital as soon as possible. During a hypertensive crisis, the condition suddenly becomes symptomatic or shows symptoms that include shortness of breath, nosebleeds, severe anxiety, and severe headaches.

THE RIGHT WAY TO TAKE BLOOD PRESSURE

Here are few pointers for taking an accurate blood pressure:

- Find a comfortable position and make sure the cuff fits perfectly on your wrist or arm during measurement. It's a good idea to lift your wrist to your heart during the measurement
- Do not smoke, drink alcohol, drink coffee, or exercise one hour before the reading
- It's a good idea to take multiple readings during one sitting. Write down the results of the monitor each time
- Follow the instructions of your BP monitor during use

ED-FRIENDLY HYPERTENSION MEDICATIONS

Now you're in a quandary – do you have ED-caused hypertension, or is your hypertension medication causing erectile dysfunction? Either way, you'll have to switch to medications that will NOT cause erectile dysfunction. Once you've done that and ED is still present, you can now safely conclude that hypertension caused your ED and establish a treatment system that focuses on that problem.

Here's a list of hypertension medications that do not have ED as a side effect:

- ACE Inhibitors
- Alpha-Blockers

- Calcium Channel Blockers
- Angiotensin II Receptor Blockers

The ones you want to avoid are Beta Blockers and Diuretics since they are most likely to cause ED.

Your doctor will determine if these drugs are appropriate for you. Keep in mind that the presence of ED is just one of the factors your physician will consider when deciding on the best medication to help with your condition. You might also have heart problems, diabetes, or other issues that need to be considered when prescribing something.

DIET AGAINST HIGH BLOOD PRESSURE

Once you've switched to an ED-friendly medication, it's time to address the hypertension itself. The great news is that hypertension can be handled further with lifestyle changes, especially a rapid shift in diet. Here are few pointers to remember:

- According to research, an abundance of salt in your diet is the primary cause of high blood pressure. The ideal amount of sodium taken in a day is 1,500 milligrams for someone with HBP.
- More potassium – opt for fruits and vegetables loaded with potassium which can help normalize your BP.
- Less Sugar – too much sugar is also forbidden for people with HBP. Note that sugar is present in many food items today, even if they're not sweet. This is why it's important to check the label and make sure that you're not consuming more sugar than you're supposed to. Fruit also contains small

amounts of sugar, so it's not a good idea to eat them en masse.
- Water – drink lots of water during the day, preferably more than your usual intake. Eight glasses a day is the recommended dose, but for the sake of safety, around ten glasses would be perfect. Studies show that drinking water before taking a bath is also an effective way of lowering your blood pressure
- Concentrate on eating fruits and vegetables instead of ill-prepared food items, including those that are prepackaged or cooked through the microwave. You also want to control the amount of meat you consume as you load your body up with base food items. Fruits are a perfect dessert choice, but your diet should be filled with leafy green vegetables for the most part.
- If you can't completely eradicate alcohol from your diet, try to limit your consumption. Males can only consume two glasses each day, while women are allowed just one glass.
- Make the conscious effort of eating fatty fish at least twice a week. Fatty fish contains high amounts of omega-three fatty acids, which can help control salt and blood pressure levels in your body. If this isn't possible, taking omega-three fatty acid supplements will do the trick.

LIFESTYLE CHANGES TO HELP WITH HYPERTENSION

Lose Weight

A common treatment for overweight people with HBP, weight loss is practically a 'cure-all' for erectile dysfunction causes. You'll find that this treatment is suggested no matter what caused your ED.

Quit Smoking

Quitting smoking is another general solution for high blood pressure and erectile dysfunction; this was already discussed at length in this book.

Exercise

A 30-minute exercise each day can help address numerous health issues, not just erectile dysfunction alone.

In conclusion, once you manage to control hypertension, your ED might fix itself, or the problem may continue. The latter usually happens because of permanent damage to the blood vessels. The body is typically capable of healing itself, but there are instances when this is no longer possible – hence the need to instantly recognize high blood pressure and address it as soon as possible. Once the damage becomes too severe, surgery is the next best option.

7

PEYRONIE'S DISEASE AND ERECTILE DYSFUNCTION

Peyronie's Disease was given a very brief description in a previous Chapter, but we'll try to discuss this condition at length in this particular one. As defined, the problem is characterized by the buildup of plaque in the penis, which causes a physical disfigurement of the organ. Usually, this leads to abnormal bending of the penis that makes it difficult for blood to pass through the vessels, hence the softness of the resulting erection.

SIGNS AND SYMPTOMS

The most obvious sign of Peyronie's Disease is the bent shape of the penis, although this isn't the only indication to be on the lookout for. Pain is also a common symptom, especially during erection. You'll find that the bend is present only during erection and seriously hampers the flexibility of the penis. Some men report that the pain eases over time, but this doesn't change the bend that occurs on the penis.

Men who suffer from scarring in the hand or foot that

impeded flexibility are also more likely to suffer from the same condition.

Note that Peyronie's Disease can descend swiftly or occur slowly, depending on the specific cause of the problem. However, if it does occur slowly, paying close attention to your penis during erection will help a great deal in preventing the condition before it becomes worse. The good news is that Peyronie's Disease is NOT an STD and, therefore, not something that you got from sexual partners. Furthermore, there are currently several ways to address the problem depending on the severity of the condition. For some lucky males, the disease goes away on its own.

CAUSES OF PEYRONIE'S DISEASE

There is no exact cause for Peyronie's Disease. According to studies, trauma is the most likely cause as the plaque buildup is essentially scar tissue. The inside of the penis suffers through a trauma that bleeds internally – which means that the male is unlikely to notice the condition. It manages to heal itself, causing an internal scar tissue buildup that blocks the blood vessels, causing difficulty in their passage during erection.

Genetics also seems to be a factor as well as the intake of specific drugs. One thing for sure, however, Peyronie's Disease is not age-driven. This means that men of all ages may be affected by the condition, whether they're in their early 20s or late 60s.

ERECTILE DYSFUNCTION (ED) AND PEYRONIE'S DISEASE (PD)

First, it's important to note that having Peyronie's Disease doesn't automatically cause Erectile Dysfunction. One doesn't follow the other, so it's perfectly possible for a male with PD to have NO erectile dysfunction issues. However, it's important to note that PD doesn't just cause ED in a physical sense. The pain can deter men from sex, but it is the insecurity leading to erectile dysfunction in men more often than not. Males who suffer from Peyronie's Disease might be reluctant to have sex or suffer from low-libido production because they're too concerned about what their partner thinks about the condition. ED resulting from psychological causes – such as those stemming from Peyronie's Disease is further discussed in this book. For this Chapter, however, you'll find out about PD and the different methods to cure the problem itself.

DIAGNOSIS AND TREATMENT FOR THE CONDITION

Once you notice any pain, bending, and discomfort on the penis, It is important to see a doctor as soon as possible to get the problem evaluated. An accurate diagnosis is important before actual treatment can be administered. Fortunately, diagnosis is not that difficult and involves the following:

- A physical examination wherein the doctor feels the hardened portion of the penis to see if there is any underlying scar tissue on its length
- • In certain circumstances, the penis may be erect for the examination, necessitating a penis-lengthening injection.
- An x-ray may also be part of the procedure to see any underlying structural or scar problems

Once Peyronie's Disease has been confirmed, the doctor

may suggest several treatment options, depending on what you feel to be the most effective for your current needs. Following are some of the most common solutions for the problem:

- First, your doctor might suggest leaving it alone since Peyronie's Disease can correct itself over time. However, the self-healing process can take as long as two years, which may not be preferable to many.
- Medications are the next option, with men prescribed different drugs depending on their specific situation. These drugs are meant to soften and eventually get rid of scar tissue. However, if the medications don't work, the next step is to make use of shots that are stronger and, therefore, more likely to produce results.
- The last and least suggested method is surgery which removes the plaque and replaces it with a tissue graft. As with many surgeries, this particular method comes with several risks, including the possibility that the condition will come back. In some cases, the length of the penis may be reduced as the affected area is removed.
- A penile prosthesis can also be used where erectile dysfunction has become a problem. Penile prosthesis is further explained in this book, how it works, and who would best use this solution to help with their ED.

8

SUBSTANCE ABUSE AND ERECTILE DYSFUNCTION

Substance may refer to a lot of things in relation to erectile dysfunction. The most common forms of substance abused which lead to ED include: alcohol, cigarettes, and recreational drugs. This Chapter will attempt to tackle each of these substances and how they affect the male's capacity to perform.

ALCOHOL

Alcohol is by far the most significant substance that can affect erectile ability, mainly because there are no legal limits on how many a man can consume. Now, there are two instances when drinking alcohol can lead to ED. First is when a man is completely drunk, having imbibed enough alcohol to make sexual function impossible. However, this situation is usually temporary as erectile capability comes back after the alcohol has been flushed out of the male's system.

A common question here is: how much alcohol must a man drink before they completely lose the ability to perform? This depends largely on the tolerance of the male. Alcoholics have a higher tolerance built over time, while others may have a lower threshold. It would be difficult to give a specific amount that will apply to everyone.

However, the second type of ED refers to alcoholics or those who consume large amounts of alcohol regularly. Constant imbibing of alcohol can lead to several complications, damaging the liver, causing issues with the nerves, relaxing the muscles too much, affecting the brain, and even lowering the amount of libido a person has. If you find yourself drinking massive amounts of alcohol daily and suffering from ED, it is advisable to stop drinking entirely.

Now: how long should one detoxify from alcohol before regaining erectile function? Much like the first question, the answer to this is indefinite. For sure, alcoholics will experience a rapid decline in their sexual activity – this could take a few months or even a year to become obvious. In most cases, even an alcoholic who happens to be sober will have difficulty maintaining an erection.

Solving the Issue

If you feel as though alcohol is the primary reason for your ED, there is no other way to stop rather than simply quitting alcohol intake. Opt for a cold turkey approach instead of simply cutting back on the amount you consume daily.

CIGARETTES

Studies show that there's a direct relationship between smoking cigarettes and erectile dysfunction. Long-term smoking causes plaque buildup of the vessels, making it difficult for the blood to flow through the shaft. This results in insufficient hardness during erection, making it near impossible to perform penetration.

The positive news is that plaque buildup does not last forever. You should be able to cure ED by stopping smoking and giving your body the chance to 'clean' itself without exposing it to more nicotine. The positive news is that nicotine is finally washed out of your system 48 hours after the last cigarette. However, it might take longer if you're the type who smokes several cigarettes in a single day. To have the greatest performance, you can abstain from cigarettes for at least four weeks to see if it affects your erectile dysfunction.

Flushing Nicotine Faster

Lifestyle and emotional factors may slow down the process of nicotine flushing. Note that just because you've quit smoking doesn't mean you'll be able to regain your normal sexual function. The determining factor here is nicotine which means that if you're using nicotine patches or nicotine gum to quit, you're not flushing out the substance out of your body. You're simply lowering the amount of your intake with the goal of completely banning the substance. If this is your preferred path towards the goal, then this shouldn't be a problem. Note, though, that you should start counting the days after your last exposure to nicotine.

Here are some suggestions for quickening the nicotine flushing process:

- Drink lots of water every day – nicotine is water-soluble, which means that with sufficient amounts of water in your system, the flushing process becomes faster
- Exercise is also a great way to start shedding the

nicotine in your body. It speeds up metabolism and allows nicotine to be flushed out through sweat
- You can also start taking vitamin C supplements to boost your metabolism. Studies show that nicotine fights with vitamin C and manages to destroy it, which can be bad for your health. With a steady supply, you'll be able to regain your health and prevent any possible side effects of nicotine – including erectile dysfunction

RECREATIONAL DRUGS

Recreational drugs may include cocaine, marijuana, heroin, and even ED medication. The above implies that men who have been used to Viagra before sex grow a dependency that renders it impossible for them to achieve an erection normally. The link between ED and recreational drugs is hardly surprising, considering how recreational drugs affect every possible aspect of a person's body. It inhibits blood flow, can cause damage to the brain, blood vessels, and essentially every other organ – including the penis. In cases like this, there is no other option but to stop the intake of recreational drugs to hopefully alleviate erectile dysfunction problems.

Note that there are 'points of no return' when it comes to ED caused by recreational drug use. This means that the damage has become so extensive that the body is no longer capable of initiating the healing process all on its own. In cases like these, medical intervention becomes necessary.

STEROIDS

Steroids occupy a special paragraph all on their own because many men take for granted the extent of their impact on daily use. Steroids are used for muscle-building purposes. It manages to boost testosterone production, hence the sudden speed in the development of muscles. When used excessively, however, steroids can cause fluctuations in hormone production which leads to erectile dysfunction. Not only that, but the condition can also decrease sex drive and bring on mood swings for many men. Additional side effects of steroid use include liver damage and even infertility. Once you stop, however, and no permanent damage has set in, there's a good chance that the erectile dysfunction will cure itself.

9

SEXUALLY TRANSMITTED DISEASES (STD) AND ERECTILE DYSFUNCTION

Sexually Transmitted Diseases or STD may also cause erectile dysfunction. Now, you probably think that ED itself is a type of STD, but this is far from the truth. More often than not, ED is a symptom of an STD which means that you'll have to address the STD first with the hope that the ED will follow through.

HOW STDS CAUSE ED

The most prevalent question here is: exactly what STD causes erectile dysfunction? The truth is that on a psychological level – all of them can. From syphilis to Chlamydia – all these diseases can trigger sufficient depression to affect the male's ability to perform in bed.

Physically speaking, STDs can also discourage men from attaining an erection. This is because many STDs cause pain to the penis, whether flaccid or erect. The pain is often enough distraction to dampen the male enthusiasm towards sex.

As a direct result of the STD, however, erectile dysfunction isn't usually a symptom. For many men, what could lead to STD is infertility or the impossibility of having children. For this reason, it's important to constantly have your sexual health checked to ensure that you have zero STD. This is especially true for men who have multiple sexual partners.

STD DIAGNOSIS AND TREATMENT

Sexually transmitted diseases are more likely in males who have multiple sexual partners. For the most part, ED-caused STD occurs when the STD is already in the severe stage. However, you shouldn't wait 'for this to occur before having yourself checked, especially if you've had sex with more than one woman for the past few months.

STD checks are pretty routine, including a physical checkup, questions asked, and samples requested of urine, semen, or blood. It's best to have yourself checked for STD frequently if you have more than one sexual partner in months or feel any signs of symptoms involving your sexual organ.

10
PORNOGRAPHY AND ERECTILE DYSFUNCTION

Studies show that the abundance of pornography and its frequent use also has an effect on male sexual performance. More particularly, it lowers libido – thereby making it hard for men to maintain arousal during actual sex with a partner.

According to experts, instances of porn-induced ED are more common than other people realize. Males who are 15 years of age up to their late 20s are the most common individuals who report having the condition. Statistically speaking, 15 to 20 percent of men who go to doctors for ED do so because of the overconsumption of porn.

SIGNS OF PORN OVERCONSUMPTION ERECTILE DYSFUNCTION

So how do you know if your erectile dysfunction stems from this particular condition? Following are some of the risk factors and symptoms associated:

- Watching porn daily

- Using porn to masturbate on a daily or several times a week
- Having difficulty obtaining an erection or maintaining one during sex with a partner even though you are more than eager to perform
- Very little difficulty in maintaining an erection while watching porn
- You don't have any morning wood, or you don't suffer from any kind of sudden or spontaneous erection
- Difficulty in reaching orgasm when with a real girl
- You might have to escalate porn watching to achieve orgasm. For example, you find yourself switching to a different genre that you don't really like
- There are no other physical problems that could trigger erectile dysfunction
- Even enhancement drugs have zero effect on you in terms of satisfaction

Hence, young males who don't suffer from diabetes, cardiovascular diseases, or any other health issues but still have ED might have porn-induced problems. This occurs because daily doses of porn condition your sexual preferences, programming your mind to become aroused at very specific stimuli triggers – such as images on the computer and your hand wrapped around your member.

This can also cause unrealistic expectations in males, especially when it comes to female reactions. Men who have become accustomed to watching specific porn with specific women and expecting a certain reaction might struggle when confronted with the real thing.

How Do You Check?

So how can you tell exactly that porn is the cause of your erectile dysfunction? Try this:

1. Masturbate without using any other stimulation but your imagination. Imagine yourself with a girl you like and thinking about regular sex. Do this in a relaxed environment such as your bedroom, and don't force the sensation. Use a relaxed grip on your penis and see if you can obtain an erection or reach an orgasm using this technique.
2. If you had problems getting an erection or failed to have one completely, try it for the second time – this time using porn as your sexual stimuli. If this time, there's virtually no difficulty to the process, this is as good as a confirmation of having porn-related ED.

SOLVING PORN-RELATED ED

The good news is that porn-related ED is curable – but you'll need more than just Viagra or medications to make it possible. In this instance, the issue is psychological – the penis is perfectly capable, but the brain is not providing the necessary trigger. More often than not, the process involves a 12-step program that slowly reconditions the brain so that it once again responds to the normal sexual stimuli. Here's how it works: Porn Addiction

First things first, it's important to know if you're addicted to porn. If you are, we'll have to address the addiction first before pursuing the need to treat erectile dysfunction. If you answered YES to over three of these questions, you're a lifestyle addict:

1. Do you suddenly have an increased tolerance for

porn? For example, have you ventured to more hardcore genres to get a reaction?
2. Do you find yourself craving porn for sexual release?
3. Do you mentally commit to watching porn for just a few minutes but find yourself spending more time on the activity?
4. Do you postpone important activities to watch porn?
5. Do you devote a significant amount of time, energy, internet access, and data storage to porn?
6. Have you tried to reduce your porn consumption or quit completely but failed to do so?

COLD TURKEY APPROACH

When quitting smoking, drinking, or whatever addiction, the 'slow but sure' approach is usually recommended. The idea is that it allows your body to gradually recalibrate its system so that you won't have to suffer from all the 'withdrawal' symptoms.

However, the same approach does NOT work for curing erectile dysfunction. All men who were brave enough to come upfront about their Porn-Induced Erectile Dysfunction (PIED) noted that kicking the habit down a notch doesn't do anything. In fact, it only 'rewires' the brain so that now, instead of being turned on by pornography, you find yourself getting turned on by erotica or literary porn.

The best way to go, therefore, is the cold turkey approach. The goal is simple: to go as many days as you can without masturbating, watching porn, imagining sexual acts, looking at pornographic images, reading erotic materials, or even actually having sex with a partner.

Why Cold Turkey?

The cold turkey approach essentially helps your mind recalibrate to its original setting of what causes arousal. This refers to the natural movement of the body, the feel of actual skin on your skin, the sounds, and the response of your partner. Now – it might take a long time to recover using the Cold Turkey approach, and to be honest, there's no specific 'timeline' between deciding to stop watching porn and complete recovery. However, it is strongly advised that you do NOT masturbate, watch porn, or even imagine having sex during such time. Now, this might be tough, especially if you're used to the activity, but just think of the positive consequences afterward:

- The ability to fully enjoy yourself again during sex with a woman
- The capacity to have and maintain an erection
- Morning wood or unexpected erections return

SUGGESTED STEPS FOR RECOVERY

Step 1

Just stop watching porn and masturbating to it. This includes all types of erotic material, including still images and erotica.

Step 2

One month after not doing anything sexual, you can start masturbating again WITHOUT using any other stimuli but your hand and your imagination. If you feel like setting the mood first, like taking a bath or lighting some candles, then feel free to do your thing as long as it doesn't involve any sort of porn.

Remember, one month is the minimum amount of time that you should wait. If your efforts after one month aren't working, then chances are you need a longer time to 'detoxify' from the condition.

Note that you don't have to masturbate daily. In fact, that's discouraged. Ideally, masturbation should only be done 2 to 3 times per week as your schedule permits.

Step 3

During masturbation, you're achieving two things: arousal of the penis and ejaculation. In Step 3, you'd want to make sure that you're not just capable of achieving orgasm but can sustain the erection for a long period – enough to keep your partner satisfied.

This exercise is common among men and utilized to help with premature ejaculation and generally improve your bed performance. Start by masturbating and achieving hardness sufficient for penetration. However, do NOT allow yourself to ejaculate or reach orgasm just yet.

Once you get hard, try counting to ten and see if you remain hard all through this time. If you do, count to twenty next time. If your penis starts to soften before reaching the count of ten, repeat the exercise until you remain hard throughout the count.

Repeat Step 3 several times in 4 weeks, each time increasing your count on how long you can stay hard.

Step 4

Now it's time to mimic real sex – without the partner.

Now, that might sound weird, but the truth is that during Step 4, you'll simply try changing positions during masturbation. You can be on your back, sitting down, on all fours, or standing up. Try masturbating while assuming the typical positions males have during actual sex with a lady. This is done so that you stop associating sitting down to watch porn as the only way to get off.

You can even put on a condom, get yourself properly aroused, switch positions, and continue masturbating – going for as long as necessary until you're ready to ejaculate. All the while, your penis should remain hard.

Once you've managed to go through each step, you're probably ready to get back to real sex with real ladies instead of something inspired by porn. If that doesn't work, it's time to check in with a therapist. For the most part, however, this technique should give you back your past sexual experience. Remember: once you've got your old virility back, don't regress to porn.

11

CONFIDENCE AND SELF-TALK – THE PSYCHOLOGICAL SIDE OF ERECTILE DYSFUNCTION

Psychological reasons may also be the cause of ED, in which case, therapy is the most likely treatment. Due to the sensitive nature of the cause, however, one cannot instantly be prescribed treatment without first understanding the full extent of Psychological Erectile Dysfunction (PED).

CAUSES OF PSYCHOLOGICAL ERECTILE DYSFUNCTION

There are two core reasons why PED might occur. Although they may seem simple at first, the truth is that these two categories can be further divided into subcategories:

- Stress and Anxiety – Stress and anxiety may be caused by numerous events in a person's life, starting from work, family life, relationships, or even insomnia. Study shows that lack of sleep – especially consistently – is sufficient to cause stress levels that can lead to erectile dysfunction.
- Depression – loss of a loved one, loss of

employment, relationship problems, and sometimes hormonal imbalance can cause depression, leading to ED. Depression tends to lower libido and desire, which makes it near impossible for the male to perform.

Which Came First?

Chances are your PED stems from these two categories after suffering through a major depressive or stress-inducing moment in your life. As previously discussed, what's tricky about PED is that it feeds on itself. For example, you're currently stressed so that when your partner initiates sex, you are unable to obtain an erection. Say this happened two or three times. Fear and shame over not being able to compete sexually will build up over time, making you doubt your desire to have sex.

So now it's important to ask yourself: are you unable to perform because you're stressed, or are you stressed because you're not able to perform? If the answer is the latter, then you may consider this a one-off problem that can be addressed by de-stressing yourself. However, if it is the former, we'll have to delve deeper into what is causing the stress and go from there.

TIPS TO HANDLE STRESS AND ANXIETY

Take a Vacation from Sex

People unwind in different ways, but for ED, it's usually best to simply stop dwelling about your non-performance in bed. Don't force yourself into having sex because you'll only feel worse about yourself each time you have difficulty maintaining an erection. That being said, practice celibacy for a few days, weeks, or even a month.

De-Stress

With your focus gone from sexual dysfunction, it's time to handle the stress issue. Now, there are several ways for people to unwind, and the effectiveness may vary depending on what you're most receptive about. That being said, it's suggested that you simply focus on things that help you relax. Following are some items that could help:

- Eat correctly – a high diet of fast foods, fried dishes, and junk food will only promote anxiety and depression. Try to focus on eating healthy, which includes fish, fruits, and vegetables
- Exercise is one of the most effective forms of de-stressing. Go to the gym or take a leisurely walk at the beach, in the forest, or wherever you feel most at ease
- It's also possible to de-stress with several friends. Make it a night out with them or even a weekend, depending on your preferences
- Take good long sleep. Studies show that sleep has a way of 'rebooting' the mind and allowing the body to relax completely.
- Take up meditation which helps lower the levels of stress-causing hormones while at the same time sharpening your mind and enhancing memory

Masturbate and Enjoy

Now, completely removing stress and anxiety from your person will not happen overnight – but you'll be able to accurately judge when you're ready to get back in the game. There's no rush here: your first try would be an incredible mood booster, so it's crucial that you manage to get a significant leap in improvement.

Ideally, your first try should NOT be with a woman. Instead, it's best to take your time and masturbate. You have the option to use porn or simply use your imagination to make things work. What's important, however, is that you DO NOT rush things. Find a comfortable place and time for the activity and choose the scenario that works best for your arousal.

Remember: the goal here is not to ejaculate as fast as you can but rather be able to sustain the pleasure long enough for a decent erection. Try to delay your ejaculation for as long as possible. In this manner, you are essentially participating in Jelqing, a common exercise used to help with Erectile Dysfunction. More on Jelqing will be discussed later.

RELATIONSHIP PROBLEMS

When it comes to PED, relationship issues fall under the category of Stress and Anxiety, but they require their own discussion. Problems in the relationship leading to ED are often confined in the bedroom wherein the male initiates sexual relations, and the partner rejects the advances. Should this occur often – or even just once – the male's ability to muster confidence for sex becomes compromised.

The male's inability to offer the female sexual satisfaction is also another root of erectile dysfunction. It is not uncommon for certain men to have premature ejaculation issues, which progress to erectile dysfunction when they feel the weight and discomfort of not being able to perform properly in bed.

Psychological issues such as these are not easy to tackle,

especially since it involves two people instead of just one. If you feel any insecurity in the relationship stemming from sexual performance, addressing the issue alone won't be as effective as talking about it as a couple.

That being said, erectile dysfunction stemming from relationship problems is best addressed through sexual therapy.

TIPS TO HANDLE DEPRESSION – ERECTILE DYSFUNCTION

What if your ED stems from depression rather than stress and anxiety? It is necessary to remember that depression is a more serious condition that necessitates a multifaceted approach to treatment. In order to cure ED, you'll have to address the cause of depression itself and go from there. Here's how you handle the depression:

- Seek out a therapist to assist you with your depression.
- The use of anti-depressants can also help alleviate the negative emotions impacting erectile dysfunction
- Take a vacation or look for methods to relieve yourself of stress and anxiety. For most, even a single step towards cheering yourself up can help with the depressive mood
- Another tried-and-true approach is to be surrounded by friends and relatives.

CONFIDENCE BOOSTER

The great thing about PED is that you can feed on your initial confidence to ensure that erectile dysfunction won't happen again. For example, if you've managed to successfully have sex with your partner once, you can rely on this previous success to accomplish a second, a third, a fourth, or an nth session with your significant other.

Now, it might seem 'cliché' to say that you only need to 'feel confident' about yourself to successfully initiate sex – but the truth is that this is where it starts. To avoid disappointing yourself, you must think of yourself as someone who will follow through with intimacy.

Now, there are several ways you can boost your confidence in preparation for sex. Most men like to work out – the improvement in their physique giving the necessary assurance to make them happy about themselves. Others like to relax, while others may choose to engage in a preparatory ritual designed to make them feel more confident.

One highly useful confidence-booster however, is encouragement from your partner. Males who have a partner willing to get them excited and offering encouragement can help ensure that there is no insecurity in the bedroom. Unfortunately, such cannot be achieved without some cooperation from the other party – hence the need for sexual therapy.

SEX THERAPY

Sex Therapy is by far the most approved treatment when it comes to PED. Note though that Sex Therapy is different from the therapy undertaken for depression that causes erectile dysfunction. Through Sex Therapy, you'll be given a more refined approach to Erectile Dysfunction and how to get your sexual health back on track.

How Sex Therapy Works

It's important to note that Sex Therapy is a wide-ranging treatment that doesn't just cover males who suffer from erectile dysfunction. For the purposes of this book, however, Sex Therapy targets the possible underlying reasons for ED and how it can be solved. For the most part, a Sex Therapist tackles several topics with their patient, including but not limited to the following:

- Possible psychological factors relating to ED
- The events that led to the ED
- What the patient thinks or feels about their ED situation
- How the patient views themselves with the ED problem
- Any questions or frustrations the patient might have about ED and how it affects their sex life
- An evaluation of the different treatments made available for ED and what would be the best choice possible
- Sex Therapists also become involved when patients are about to undergo serious treatments for ED, particularly those that are surgical in nature

Finding a Therapist

The positive thing is that there are many Sex Therapists available nowadays. For the most part, you should go with the recommendation of your GP or the doctor specially tasked to help with ED. Some factors to consider when finding your Sex Therapist include:

- Start by checking the AASECT or the American Association of Sexuality Educators, Counselors, and Therapists. This should provide you with a reliable list of possible sex therapists in your area.

- It's also possible to ask trusted friends, families, or doctors for a recommendation
- Find more about the credentials of the sex therapist. This includes license, what school they graduated in, and the years of experience they've had in the job. References are also a perfect way to learn more about the individual you've picked.
- Lastly, have a preliminary consult – preferably at no expense to you. Sex therapy is a deeply personal treatment requiring trust between you and your therapist. That being said, it's crucial that you feel at ease or comfortable with the person you're talking to.

Success Rate

Sex Therapy has a proven success record. Unfortunately, not many men are willing to undergo therapy for the simple reason that they feel awkward talking about their sex life. However, keep in mind that Sex Therapists are specially trained to handle any sexual issue their patients might have, including but not limited to Erectile Dysfunction.

According to studies, men who seek Sex Therapy with their respective partners achieve better results than those who choose to keep their sessions private.

HOW TO BRING THE EXCITEMENT BACK IN SEX

Now – some men would want to try every possible avenue before seeking the help of a sex therapist, which makes sense if your insurance doesn't cover this particular need. Here's how you can slowly ignite the spark in your relationship and hopefully bypass the psychological dilemma of erectile dysfunction:

- Go high tech with foreplay, starting with sexy texts or chats, telling her exactly what you intend to do when you finally get home. Send nude selfies if that's your thing – just make sure all the information you send remains private.
- Build the anticipation with prolonged foreplay. Set the stage and make good use of sexy aphrodisiacs to get you started. Incorporating food into the equation can be extremely sexy, with chocolate, wine, and strawberries being some of the best options today.
- Turn it into a game, allowing her to play as much as she would want with your body or vice versa. You can act out various sexual fantasies such as being tied down or wearing a blindfold
- Sex toys are also a great way to boost the excitement in the bedroom. Make sure she gives her approval before doing anything.
- Have fun when it comes to position. Rent a Kama Sutra video if you have to and just run with it.

IMPORTANT: keep in mind that leveling up the sex is a double-edged sword. For example, men who find themselves having a penchant for sex toys may no longer be aroused if such toys are no longer part of intimacy. Hence, it's important to take a few steps back after sizzling up the bedroom so that you'll still be able to enjoy sex in its most basic version.

12

NON-SURGICAL ED TREATMENTS – DEVICE AND MEDICATIONS

Of course, there are instances when changing your diet and exercise routine just won't cut it. Short of undergoing surgical treatments for erectile dysfunction, it's always possible to opt for the use of devices. The good news is that there are many of them on the market, each one perfect depending on the cause of your ED. Here are only a few ideas for you to try right now: Vacuum Constriction Devices are a form of vacuum constriction device.

VACUUM CONSTRICTION DEVICES

Often used by males who have ED due to diabetes, a vacuum constriction device comprises a pump and a band. The penis is placed inside the pump with the band wrapped around the root of the penis, the two working together to help achieve and maintain the hardness of an erection.

How It Works

- Start by putting the penis inside the pump

- Start pumping the air out of the container using the attachment at the top of the cylinder. This should promote blood flow to the penis, causing it to become harder and erect.
- Once the penis is fully erect, grab a lubricant and slowly slide the retaining band to the bottom part of the penis. There is no need to do this fast – your main concern is to ensure that the shaft remains hard without causing any injury.
- Release the vacuum and remove the pump
- Most males attempt intercourse afterward, keeping the constricting band in place. This helps maintain the erection and 'train' the nerves into once again accommodating blood flow and keeping it.
- It might take 3 or 4 times of practice before you can get the hang of using a VCD. It's advisable to practice this at least two times a day to see if you can achieve hardness sufficient for penetration.

There are currently dozens of VCD products in the market today, but go with what your doctor has prescribed. When buying one, however, one important feature to look for is the 'quick release' option which lets you release the vacuum when needed. Injury is possible if the vacuum isn't released quickly enough or within the specified time. Generally, all VCD's operate the same way, but it's best to follow your product's instructions to the letter, especially when it comes to the amount of time you can keep your penis in the vacuum.

Effectiveness and Safety

As already mentioned, VCDs are relatively safe, provided that they have a quick-release function for the vacuum. Other than this and with proper use, you shouldn't have any problems with VCD. As for effectiveness, studies show that an average of 8 out of 10 men finds it effective, offering sufficient hardness for penetration. Note though that you should NOT use this too often as some problems might occur. Common side effects of frequent or improper use include: bruising, pinched scrotal tissue, tenderness, numbness, pain, and sensitivity. If any of these conditions appear, try not to use the VCD for several days and resume only when you're feeling well again.

Who Should Use It?

VCDs are best used by males who suffer from diabetes or poor blood flow to the penis. If you suffer from any other condition leading to erectile dysfunction, it's best to consult your doctor beforehand about the use of VCD.

Note that VCD-erections may feel slightly different from normal erections, so you might want to talk to your partner before using this method for intercourse.

ERECTILE DYSFUNCTION RINGS

ED Rings are also a common tool used for ED problems. They're essential 'rings' that are inserted in the penis and lodged along with the roots, essentially constricting the base so that the erection remains.

How it Works

ED rings work by preventing the blood from flowing backward out of the penis. Imagine wrapping a band around the base of your finger, causing the blood to pool into that one particular area. This is essentially how ED rings work but at a gentler state to not damage the blood vessels. To use ED rings, here's what you should do:

- Start by attaining an erection through any means you feel necessary, such as pumps or straightforward masturbation.
- Once you've achieved a hardness conducive for penetration, lubricate the ED ring and gently slip it to the base of the penis
- Check that the ring does not trap any pubic hair or scrotal tissue, as this may trigger pinching.

At this point, the ED ring will now help you maintain that erection long enough for intercourse. Some men simply use ED rings for 'practice,' allowing their shaft to get used to the sensation and essentially treating ED at a leisurely pace.

Effectiveness and Safety

ED rings are remarkably safe, considering that they're easy to put on and remove. As with most penile products, however, it's crucial to follow the instructions of their use; otherwise, you might find yourself having issues. Bruising, discomfort, and tenderness are common problems with ED rings for first-time users. As for effectiveness, studies show that 80% of men who use this are happy with the results. It's interesting to note that even males who don't suffer from ED use these rings to boost their performance.

Who Should Use It?

If you notice, ED rings are no different from the rings used during VCDs. When it comes down to it, there is no discernible distinction between the two – VCD rings are simply those that are accompanied by pumps used to stimulate erection. Independent ED rings are those used by men who can achieve erection WITHOUT the help of the pump or vacuum.

INTRAURETHRAL THERAPY

Intraurethral therapy is another common treatment for ED, often administered at home. There are two ways of achieving an erection through this method: injection or pellets. Through the administration of the drug, the penis manages to achieve sufficient erection for intercourse.

How it Works

One of the reasons males are doubtful about this method is because intraurethral therapy addresses the penis directly. The drug – usually alprostadil – is injected into the penis specifically, which can be a bit awkward for males. Hence, if you have problems with needles, it's best to use the pellet version of this particular ED medication.

Effectiveness and Safety

In terms of effectiveness, there's no question that intraurethral therapy does its job perfectly. Nearly 100% of men who try this method achieve an erection sufficient for penetration. Users note that the product takes effect 10 to 15minutes after administration, so it's best to use it before intercourse. Note though that despite the effectiveness of the product, there are some problems that may surface:

- Pain, usually resulting from improper introduction of the drug into the penis

- Priapism, a condition wherein the penis abnormally maintains an erection of at least 4 hours. When this occurs, damage may happen to the blood vessels of the penis, thereby requiring medical attention.

Who Should Use It?

Intraurethral therapy is best used by men who have diabetes or vascular problems resulting in erectile dysfunction. Note that intraurethral therapy is not a cure for ED and must be used before every intercourse.

VIAGRA

Viagra is perhaps the most popular medication for Erectile Dysfunction nowadays. Also known as those little blue pills, Viagra can work wonders and has been known to take effect among the majority of its users. The drug often works for 4 hours.

Intake

Viagra is a prescribed drug which means that you'll have to follow the exact instructions provided by your doctor. It's best to take 30 minutes before any sexual interaction to ensure effectiveness.

Warning

Viagra should NOT be taken along with any nitrate drug usually used for cardiovascular issues. Intake of nitrate along with Viagra can result in blood pressure issues. Ensure your doctor about any health problems and medication you're taking so that they'd know whether Viagra is the right ED for you.

Side Effects

It's important to distinguish between common side effects and those that should lead you to contact the doctor. Flushing, headache, abnormal vision, dizziness, stuffy nose, back pain, muscle pain, and upset stomach are just some of the drug's common side effects. However, the emergence of any of the following requires medical intervention:

- Swelling of hands and ankles
- Irregular heartbeat
- Pain and pressure on the chest
- Vision changes or vision loss
- An erection that is painful or lasts more than four hours
- Hearing loss or abnormal hearing
- Shortness of breath
- Seizure
- Lightheaded feeling

CIALIS

Cialis works significantly longer compared to Viagra. In fact, some instances reveal that Cialis works up to 36 hours, making it ideal for many men. Like Viagra, Cialis doesn't instantly produce an erection after intake. A male has to be aroused in order for an erection to occur, which can happen multiple times during the course of the affectivity of the medication.

Intake

Cialis is best taken roughly 30 minutes before any sexual activity. The initial dose is set at 10mg orally, but any following doses are reduced to just 5mg for Erectile Dysfunction. The product is used as needed, but there are those who take the item daily but reduce it to just 2.5mg to ensure performance each time intimacy is initiated.

Warning

Alcohol is generally prohibited when taking any kind of medication. Grapefruit juice and other citrus fruits are also discouraged when taking Cialis because it can produce adverse reactions. If you have any of the above health problems or are taking medicine for them, make sure to inquire or tell your doctor ahead of time:

- Heart problems
- Bleeding disorder
- Stomach ulcer
- Kidney problems
- Liver disease
- Angina
- Stroke
- Deformity of the penis

Side Effects

Common side effects of the medication include sore throat, sinus pain, headache, and muscle pain. Signs of an allergic reaction, including hives, swelling of the tongue, lips, throat, or face, and difficulty breathing, should be looked at immediately by a doctor. Side effects that are uncommon and require medical intervention include but are not limited to the following:

- An erection that lasts over four hours
- Painful erection
- Changes in vision
- Ear ringing or hearing loss
- Chest pain or pressure
- Irregular heartbeat
- Shortness of breath
- Seizure
- Swelling of the hands or feet
- Lightheadedness

LEVITRA

Another common medication for erectile dysfunction, Levitra, works by relaxing the muscles around the vessels, resulting in an impressive and strong erection.

Intake

Levitra is taken orally with a limit of just 20 mg per day. Ordinarily, however, the initial dose is set at 10mg, followed by 5mg for maintenance purposes. Note that Levitra should be taken as needed upon which it will remain effective for the next 4 to 5 hours when the male is aroused. Do NOT take Levitra more than once a day – it's crucial to let 24 hours pass before your second intake; otherwise, it can take its toll on the body.

Warning

Do not take Levitra and alcohol at the same time or consecutively. Grapefruit and other citrus products should also be avoided. Generally speaking, patients must inform their doctor if they suffer from health conditions or taking any sort of medication. The following health issues or medications to treat the issues must not coexist with Levitra use:

- Heart disease
- Blood pressure issues
- Seizure
- Liver or Kidney disease
- Bleeding disorder
- Stomach ulcer
- Hearing and vision problems
- Deformity of the penis

Side Effects

Levitra is likely to produce an allergic reaction in some individuals comprised of hives, itching, and swelling. If you experience some of these symptoms after taking Levitra, see a medical professional immediately! Common side effects that shouldn't worry you too much are: back pain, flushing, headache, dizziness, stuffy nose, and upset stomach. The following symptoms, however, need to be taken more seriously:

- Visio changes
- Ringing in ears or hearing loss
- Pain or pressure on the chest
- Swelling of the hands or feet
- Shortness of breath
- Painful erection
- An erection that lasts over four hours
- Feeling of passing out
- Irregular heartbeat
- Convulsions or seizures

13

SURGICAL TREATMENTS FOR ERECTILE DYSFUNCTION

Surgical treatments for ED should be a last resort for males, considering how the process can be painful and requires long-term recovery. The good news is that surgical procedures are becoming more popular among physicians who have the medical know-how and experience to guarantee success after the operation. Today, you'll find several surgical treatments for Erectile Dysfunction: Vascular Reconstructive Surgery

VASCULAR RECONSTRUCTIVE SURGERY

As the name suggests, this surgery involves reconstructing the vessels to boost or improve blood flow to the penis. The goal is to clear arteries so that the bloodflow to the penis is uninterrupted, ensuring a harder erection. It functions by moving an artery from the stomach to the penis, increasing blood flow to the organ.

Due to the sensitivity of the surgery, however, very few doctors recommend it to older patients. In fact, Vascular Reconstructive Surgery is best used by younger males who suffer from ED due to injuries or accidents. Those who have ED because of diabetes, heart problems, hypertension, and the like are advised against this particular treatment.

Does It Work?

The surgery is not a foolproof method for beating ED. In fact, only 1 out of 20 patients seem to get long-term benefits from the operation. This is why many doctors see this as a last-ditch effort for males. On top of that, the procedure is costly and requires long-term recovery before a male can test out whether their ED is cured.

PENILE PROSTHESIS

A penile prosthesis is not exactly a new concept, with many men already sporting this type of attachment to help with their sex life. There are two types of penile prosthesis today: the 3-piece and the 2-piece. Regardless of which you choose, they work pretty much the same way.

How It Works

Prosthesis is placed through surgery in the penis, the scrotal sack, and the abdomen, depending on the type of penile implant you're getting. To cause an erection, a pump which is located discreetly in the scrotum is pressed. When finished, the same pump can be deflated so that the penis goes back to its flaccid state. The surgery is discreet enough that there is no visible evidence of any pump or material implanted into the penis or scrotum. A small scar might be visible, but your sexual partner will not be able to see much of a difference compared to a regular penis. Hence, it should not cause any embarrassment during sex or when in a locker room.

Pleasure and Use

Sex-wise, the prosthesis doesn't radically change the way a man feels during penetration. According to those who had the surgery, the duration of erection is shorter, but new developments today have easily solved this problem. The sensation on the skin and even reaching an orgasm is no different for the male.

Safety and Other Consequences

According to statistics, 95% of men who undergo penile prosthesis surgery are happy with the results and glad that they underwent the procedure. Of course, side effects are also present, although they are not that common among patients.

Some of the side effects to consider include:

- Infection
- Formation of scar tissue
- Bleeding after surgery that may require another operation
- Erosion of tissue around the implant, therefore needing removal
- Mechanical failure which leads to removal and new implant

Ideal Patients and Insurance

Penile prosthesis can be expensive, but the good news is that they are sometimes covered by insurance. Of course, this is following the assumption that the medical reason for the ED is well-established for the individual concerned.

Remember that this is a last-resort option, and should you wish to undergo the procedure, it's best to first find out the extent of insurance coverage offered. You'll find that penile implants are mainly used by men who suffer from Peyronie's Disease or those who are unlikely to recover from ED through other means. Permanent injury to the penis is also another likely reason for the implant to be considered.

14

KEGELS AND EXERCISES FOR OVERCOMING ED

Generally speaking, daily exercises have a significant bearing on erectile dysfunction. Exercise keeps the heart healthy, ensures proper blood flow, and relaxes the muscles – all of which are contributory to attaining and maintaining an erection. It's advisable for males with ED to focus on two general exercise categories: cardiovascular and target exercises.

Cardiovascular exercises are designed to keep the heart healthy while burning off any fat that could be clogging the arteries. This includes running, boxing, jumping jacks, jogging, or basically anything that will get you sweating with a fast-rate heartbeat.

Target exercises are made to boost the muscles. In terms of erectile dysfunction, they are perfect in helping you improve your confidence in the bedroom. By knowing that you look good naked, you'll be able to better pursue sexual relations or have the assurance that your partner is 100% happy about the intimacy.

The following, however, are more specialized forms of exercise designed to help with sexual health.

KEGEL EXERCISES

Kegel exercises are a popular technique used by both men and women. It targets the pelvic muscles utilized during sex, giving men and women better control of their sexual activities. For women, it helps tighten the vagina, while for men, it helps them attain harder erections as well as last longer in bed. Here's how you perform Kegel Exercises:

- Find a comfortable spot and sit down.
- Contract and relax your pelvic floor muscles. If you're not sure where they are, imagine yourself trying to stop urine flow. You should be able to feel specific muscles contract and relax while imagining this exercise.
- Simply repeat the contract-relax process, each time holding the contraction for 3 seconds or more. Do this several times a day whenever the opportunity presents itself
- The great thing about this exercise is that it can be performed practically anywhere and at any time. Make sure you practice the exercise several times a day and reap the benefits after a few weeks of consistency.

JELQING EXERCISE

Jelqing is another male technique designed to help you have longer-lasting erections. Essentially, it's an exercise for males who suffer from premature ejaculation, but those with Erectile Dysfunction should also have a good time trying out this method and improving their sexual expertise. Here's how you perform jelqing:

- Start by finding a safe and relaxing spot. Jelqing involves masturbation, so it stands to reason that you'd want somewhere private to perform the exercise.
- Masturbate until you're hard enough to effect ejaculation. Since ED may be a problem, it stands to reason that you might not always achieve sufficient hardness for penetration – but the inability to ejaculate and erectile dysfunction do not amount to the same thing
- Focus, therefore, on your need to ejaculate. Do you feel as though you're getting nearer to an orgasm? If so, create a circle with your thumb and pointing finger and squeeze the base of your penis with it. The goal here is to stall ejaculation for as long as you can. When you feel as though the need to ejaculate has lessened, you can start all over again and repeat the squeeze technique.
- You can do this at least three times before finally allowing yourself to ejaculate. You'll find that this particular exercise contributes largely to boosting your stamina and preventing premature ejaculation. It often aids in the blood supply to the penis, effectively widening the blood vessels to their full capacity to provide better and longer erections. Do this 3 or 4 days a week to help increase your bedtime performance.

15

DIET TYPE OPTIONS TO OVERCOME ERECTILE DYSFUNCTION

Diet has been reiterated time and time again as a solution for erectile dysfunction, but it can be tough to solve the problem if the only advice you're going to get is to 'eat healthily.' That being mentioned, this Chapter is devoted to adhering to unique diet programs that can help in the treatment of erectile dysfunction exacerbated by diabetes, elevated blood pressure, and heart problems.

DASH (DIETARY APPROACHES TO STOP HYPERTENSION) DIET

The DASH (Dietary Approaches to Stop Hypertension) Diet is highly advised for those with high blood pressure. If you suffer from hypertension, this is the best food regimen to lower your blood pressure and hopefully decrease the instances of erectile dysfunction.

What Is It?

The DASH Diet focuses on getting sufficient amounts of

nutrients while paying heed to portion control. Doctors often recommend it due to its comprehensive approach. It can be quite easy to follow because the diet doesn't just prescribe what food items to eat but also establishes a daily limit, therefore giving you a clear view of what can and cannot be done.

General Principles

Here's what you should know about the DASH Diet:

- There are two versions of the DASH Diet: the Standard Sodium and the Low Sodium. The first one limits your sodium intake to just 2,300 mg per day, while the other one lowers it to just 1,500 per day. For the sake of comparison, a regular diet contains 3,500 mg sodium per day.
- An additional limit is 2,000 calories each day. Hence – the DASH Diet requires you to eat no more than 2,000 calories each day, the sodium content of which must NOT exceed 2,300mg.

Vegetable Servings

Vegetables should be treated as a main dish rather than a side dish. Under the DASH Diet, you should consume at least four servings of a variety of vegetables daily. Try to measure each serving per cup, which means you can eat as much as 1 cup of vegetables during breakfast. Leafy green vegetables are the best kind when it comes to high blood pressure. Note that fresh and frozen vegetables are the best options, while canned vegetables should only be bought if the first two are not available. Always choose the 'low sodium' canned goods.

Dairy Servings

This includes all milk derivatives rich in vitamin D, calcium, and even protein. Now, not all dairy products are DASH Diet approved. It's important to opt for the ones that are low in fat if not completely fat-free. Two to three dairy servings every day are acceptable and should keep you well provided in terms of calcium. Those that are lactose intolerant should try a lactase medicine that is available over the counter – this will help you digest lactose better. Yogurt is by far the most flexible source of dairy today and should keep you happy with the choices, especially since you can boost the flavor by adding fruit into the mix.

Nuts and Seed Servings

Since nuts and seeds are rich in calories, they should be eaten in moderation – at least 4 to 5 servings per week. They contain high amounts of potassium and magnesium, which can help against certain cancers even while lowering instances of high blood pressure. Don't be concerned about the high-fat content of nuts – this is good fat and will help fight hypertension.

Nuts can be consumed as crunchy snacks, or you can opt to add them to your salad, putting a whole new dimension to leafy green as you feel a satisfying crunch with each bite.

Fruit Servings

The DASH Diet is ideal for those with hypertension and NOT with diabetes because it recommends up to 5 servings of fruit each day. Despite the health attributes of fruit, the fact is that it contains sufficient amounts of sugar that could prove negative for a diabetic.

Fruits are wonderfully flexible in that they contain all sorts of vitamins and minerals, depending on which fruit you favor. Avoid avocado and coconuts since they tend to be high in fat, but otherwise, the fruit world is your oyster!

You may incorporate the fruit into your regular yogurt servings or just enjoy it as a treat or snack. Canned fruit and frozen fruit work too, but nothing beats fresh servings. If you're going to buy something canned, make sure it has zero or low sodium.

Meat and Fish Servings

Yes – you can eat meat on a DASH Diet, provided that they're lean rather than the fatty kind that comes cheap. This can be consumed with a max of 6 portions or fewer every day. Please note that meat and fish are interchangeable, but you should NOT eat meat alone. Fish is crucial because it supplies your body with much-needed omega-3 fatty acids, which is beneficial for practically all types of health issues.

Sweet Items

Sweets are also not entirely banned from the DASH Diet – but it makes sense to limit their serving to just five a week or less if you can manage it. The 'sweets' should also be limited to sorbet, jelly, jam, low-fat cookies, fruit juices, hard candy, etc. You can choose artificial sweeteners but don't rely on them too much. Remember: sugar has no added value, so it's mainly consumed to satisfy your sweet tooth.

Fat and Oil Servings

As mentioned, avocado is one fruit that's high in the good kind of fat, so if you want to kill two birds with one stone, this is the type to go for. Keep your fat consumption to just 2 to 3 servings every day because too much fat can lead to heart problems. Ideally, you should focus only on monounsaturated fat and avoiding large amounts of cheese, margarine, cream, eggs, and anything fried.

Everything else not mentioned in the diet should be consumed in moderation or not, including alcohol and caffeine. Note that there are instances when the food items overlap – for example, avocado contains fat which means that in some instances, they can be counted as fruits and fat – thereby allowing you to cross off TWO DASH Diet requirements in one sitting. Be mindful of these overlaps to make sure you're getting the amount you need. Check your blood pressure weekly or even daily to see if the DASH Diet is working for you. Erectile Dysfunction symptoms should decrease pursuant to better health.

MEDITERRANEAN DIET

The Mediterranean Diet (MD) is perhaps one of the most praised diets today, ranking among those best used for heart health and weight loss purposes.

What Is It?

The diet is named such because it follows the diet of people in the Mediterranean. Research shows that those who live in the Mediterranean and follow this particular system in their food regimen have lower instances of cardiovascular problems – hence the sudden interest in bringing MD to the shores of the United States. Additional perks of this diet include reduced risks of Alzheimer's, cancer, and Parkinson's.

General Principles

The best thing about this diet is that it does not force you to count calories. The General Principle is quite simple: eat as if you live in one of the countries bordering the Mediterranean, such as Greece. The diet proceeds by viewing food options as a pyramid divided into four key categories. Here's a rundown of each of them.

Primary Level – Fruits, Vegetables, Grains, Oils, Herbs, Etc

This is the Mediterranean Diet's first and most critical standard. The focus is vegetables, fruits, and grain in that particular order. Your main fare would be leady greens with fruit as the primary source of sugar. Bread is an important part of daily consumption, but it's usually whole wheat which is healthier compared to the white version, plus the fact that Greeks often skip butter and margarine – preferring their bread toasted with none of the garnishing often added in the American version. As for rice, the option is usually brown.

The importance of olive oil in the diet is also astounding, as it can be used in almost every recipe. With olive oil containing high amounts of omega-3 essential fatty acids, the addition of this further lowers heart risk issues.

Secondary Level – Fish and Seafood

The second most prevalent addition to MD is fish and other types of seafood. Fish is another good source of omega-3 fatty acids while at the same time containing vitamins, minerals, and protein necessary to keep the body well-supplied and healthy. Options such as tuna, salmon, and mackerel are perhaps the most prevalent in this particular diet.

Third Level – Poultry, Cheese, Eggs, Etc.

Dairy products, eggs, and poultry occupy the third level and should be eaten sparingly – no more than twice to three days a week in limited amounts. Keep in mind that although poultry is technically meat, it is only derived from chicken or turkey and NOT beef, pork, etc. If you're going to consume dairy, make sure you're getting the low-fat or zero-fat versions.

Meat and Sweets

Occupying the topmost portion are meats and sweets, which, in this case, make them UNDESIRABLE for those following the Mediterranean Diet. Of course, that doesn't mean that you should ban them altogether from your diet, but it stands to reason that their consumption should be limited to only the smallest amount. Once or twice a month in reasonable proportions should be enough – especially when it comes to sweets. Meat must also be lean – the fatty portion removed to make sure that it doesn't affect your cholesterol levels.

What Else?

The primary goal of the Mediterranean Diet is to make sure you only get the good kind of fat derived from fruits and vegetables. Hence, anything processed is often shunned in favor of fresh versions of food. Other considerations under this food regimen are:

- Red wine is permitted but must be limited to just one glass per day. Any other kind of alcohol is best avoided.

- Salt and sugar as seasoning is also forbidden. Greeks tend to use herbs and spices for their food which includes thyme, basil, parsley, pepper, and others
- As mentioned, olive oil is heavily used in MD with butter and regular oil limited if not completely removed from the regimen.

The Mediterranean Diet is amazing that it has gained so much popularity that there are now cookbooks focused solely on this discipline. Hence, you'll find that MD won't be as restrictive as the pyramid suggests. A few months into this particular diet and you should be able to reverse the negative effects of cardiovascular issues, including those of erectile dysfunction.

GYCEMIC INDEX

The Glycemic Index is not a diet per se but rather a guideline that helps diabetics figure out whether certain food types are compatible with their nutritional needs. If you suffer from erectile dysfunction with diabetes as the primary culprit, this particular diet will follow.

What Is It?

Also known as GI, the Glycemic Index is essentially a ranking system based on the ability of certain foods to raise glucose levels in the blood. The food items are ranked 0 to 100, with the low-GI food items generally considered the best for those suffering from diabetes. The system focuses on carbohydrate content and how long it takes to convert into glucose or sugar.

Food with a fast conversion rate naturally spikes up sugar

in the blood, while those with a low conversion rate provide a slow and steady flow of energy. This is why the GI Diet is also used by those who want to lose weight.

There are three categories to GI:

- High GI – 70 and higher
- Medium GI – 56 to 69
- Low GI – 1 to 55

You should be eating food items that are within that Low GI level with moderate amounts of Medium GI and essentially nothing of those in the High GI bracket. The question is: how do you know the GI level of the current food you're eating? The internet answers that one thing with databases is letting you enter specific food items and find out exactly where they rank in the index.

Low GI

Low GI food items generally include vegetables and whole grains. Oatmeal and bran breakfast cereals are also included in the list, as well as various fleshy fruit items.

Medium GI

Some fruits fall under the Medium GI classification, including banana, pineapple, raisins, and sweet corn. Breakfast cereals can also fall under this category, depending on their specific makeup. In truth, the lines between Low and Medium GI can be somewhat blurred, hence, the need to check and make sure which one you're getting.

High GI

High GI includes a lot of sweet items, including ice cream, hard candy, and white bread. White rice and potatoes are also included in the list. Packaged food items are generally high on the GI list and should therefore be avoided as much as possible.

Some Considerations

The main issue with the GI Diet is that it doesn't take into account portion control. It is to be understood that you will be the one exercising control over the amount of food you're eating. As a general rule, whenever you're consuming anything with a high GI, consume as little of it as possible. However, with Low GI food, you can eat as many as you want without worrying about the results too much.

AFTERWORD

Erectile dysfunction (ED) is quite a delicate subject, and many men shy away from opening up to discuss their problems. ED is very common; in fact, over 18 million men in the US are affected by ED, but other estimates say the number is almost double.

It's common to experience ED as you age, and many men will experience it at some point or another, although chronic or long-term ED isn't considered normal. Erectile dysfunction, commonly known as impotence, occurs when a male is unable to achieve or acquire an erection, preventing him from having full sex, doing, or lasting in bed.

In this book, we have been able to examine the various causes of erectile dysfunction. Each of these causes was broadly discussed chapter by chapter with possible solutions —exercises, medical and non-medical devices to cure the condition.

If you have erectile dysfunction or have been battling with the problem for a long time now, you don't have to shy away from it. It is only by facing the problem you gain sexual

AFTERWORD

confidence. The solutions contained in this book will work wonders for you. So get up your feet, be strong, and get back your confidence!

REFERENCES

- Gregory, M. (2015). Erectile Dysfunction Cure: How To Cure ED
- Naturally & Quickly and Enjoy Your Intimate Life. Gregory Moto.
- James, K. (2017). Erectile Dysfunction: The Free, Natural, Proven and
- Most Effective Way To Permanently End Erectile Dysfunction. AllPark Publishing.
- J. Bella, C. Lee, S. Carrier, F. Bénard, and B. Brock, "2015 CUA
- Practice Guidelines for Erectile Dysfunction," Canadian Urological Association (2015): 1–2.
- S. Köhler, T. McVary (2016). Contemporary Treatment of Erectile
- Dysfunction: A Clinical Guide. Springer International Publishing Switzerland.
- Trow, C. Erectile Dysfunction: Natural Cure for Impotence, Premature
- Ejaculation, and Sexual Performance.

www.ingramcontent.com/pod-product-compliance
Lightning Source LLC
Chambersburg PA
CBHW021450070526
44577CB00002B/336